# THE EFFECTIVE FAMILY MEAL PLAN

# Contents


INTRODUCTION................................................................4

CHAPTER ONE: - DEFINITION.........................................6

   Family meal time...................................................6

CHAPTER TWO: - IMPORTANCE....................................8

CHAPTER THREE-: CHALLENGES.................................13

CHAPTER FOUR: - SOLUTIONS....................................15

CONCLUSION..............................................................18

# INTRODUCTION

*"Unlocking the Power of Family Meal Time: The Effective Family Meal Plan"*

Every family has its share of problems. The challenges we face within our own families can be deeply painful. From a breaking home to quarreling kids and sibling squabbles, loss of communication and family bonds, to struggling with time constraints and busy schedules, navigating the growth and development of young children and adolescents, and even attempting to reconnect with estranged family members – these are all common struggles we encounter. But what if I told you there is one simple yet powerful tool, an engaging ritual and family tradition, that has the potential to solve many of these problems?

In the pages ahead, we will explore the transformative power of an effective family meal plan. This goes far beyond just sitting down to eat together. Join me on this journey as we delve into how family meal times can be the catalyst for positive change in any family.

Whether you are a struggling couple, a single mom or dad, a foster parent, or an elder statesperson, this guide will equip you with the tools to create a meal plan that works. It will empower you to not only cook delicious meals but also nurture the growth and development of your family in a way that aligns with your values and aspirations.

Prepare to discover the hidden powers within family meal planning and family meal time. Unlock your potential to overcome challenges and strengthen your family bonds. Together, we will embark on a journey of self-discovery, learning, and transformation.

Now, let's raise the curtains on "The Effective Meal Plan: Your Guide to Making Meals that Work" and embark on a path that will revolutionize your family's dynamics.

# Chapter One

*Family Meal Time*

# CHAPTER ONE
*Family Meal Time...*

By definition, a time when the whole family comes down to settle and eat together. Those few fractions of the day where the entirely family spends together and eats together. But, it's more than just a simple definition. It's a cherished moment, a ritual that holds the power to bring an entire family together. In those precious moments, the walls of the home come alive with laughter, conversation, and the comforting aroma of food filling the air.

Imagine the scene: a table adorned with dishes lovingly prepared, family members gathering around, their faces lighting up with anticipation. The clinking of cutlery, the sound of joyful chatter, and the shared excitement of what lies ahead. It's a symphony of togetherness, a symphony that resonates deep within our hearts.

In today's fast-paced world, finding the time and space for a proper family meal can feel like a daunting task. But amidst the chaos and demands of everyday life, carving out those sacred moments for family nourishment is more important than ever. It's a deliberate choice, a conscious commitment to prioritize the bonds that tie us together.

Why does it matter, you may ask? Because within the realm of family meal time lays a world of hidden treasures. It's a gateway to building stronger relationships, fostering deeper connections, and creating lasting memories. It's a time when parents can truly engage with their children, listening to their stories, dreams, and fears. It's an opportunity for siblings to share their triumphs and challenges, forging unbreakable bonds of support and camaraderie.

# Chapter Two

*The Power and Importance of
an Effective Meal Plan*

# CHAPTER TWO
*The Power and Importance of an Effective Meal Plan*

The importance of this little and somewhat insignificant ritual goes a long way in the life of our kids, parents and even the society we seek to develop if you ask me.

Family, they say, is first agent of socialization. The smallest unit of society. And the most powerful in nurturing bad growing how the future of a society will be. Family meal time therefore holds a special place in the hearts of families around the world. It is more than just a moment to sit down and eat together; it is a cherished tradition that brings loved ones closer, strengthens bonds, and creates lasting memories.

When the whole family gathers around the table, something magical happens. Conversations flow, laughter fills the air, and a sense of togetherness envelops everyone present. It is one of those precious moments that family members truly get a chance to connect with one another on a deeper level. They share stories, exchange ideas, and listen attentively, creating a space where every voice is heard and valued.

But the importance extends beyond the joy of being together; it also has numerous benefits for individuals and families alike. One of its remarkable aspects is its power to foster communication.

As family members engage in meaningful conversations during meals, they strengthen their ability to express themselves, actively listen, and empathize with one another. You can cultivate in your kids good speech and listening skills using this special moments. The open and honest communication around family meals is a sure way to inculcate into family and kids a supportive and understanding sense of maturity that makes them feel safe to share their thoughts, experiences, and feelings. And, more importantly, listen to others.

Give your kids chance to speak at meal tables is a very good step to improving self confidence. It's the very first stage they'll hit so let them conquer that stage fright flawlessly. By encouraging them to speak up you're not only getting them to talk and speak about themselves, but instilling good confidence and listening skills which will eventually be important as they grow into society.

Moreover, family meal time also nurtures the bonds between family members. Talking and listening, dialogue. It has always been a tool of unity and resolution of conflict. The perfect chance for talk through and listen session family meal time creates give a sense of belonging and unity, reminding everyone that they are part of something greater than themselves. As they gather around the table, they learn about each other's lives, interests, and dreams.

Amongst young kids and adolescents, foster kids and extended family. It's probably the most observable time you'll get to see them together. The shared knowledge they have during meals can help build a foundation of trust and support, strengthening the emotional connection among them as a family.

Other benefits of a good family meal plan are helping to cultivate healthy eating habits. You'd find out you're able to promote and encourage good and healthy food choices amongst kids during family meal time. When families eat together, they have the opportunity to plan and prepare nutritious meals as a team. Parents in turn serve as role models by making healthy food choices and teaching their children about balanced nutrition.

It's not a day's ask and it'll prove daunting. But its importance, not only benefits physical well-being but also instills lifelong habits that contribute to a healthier lifestyle.

Preserving cultural and family values. Culture is a way of life, an ancestry, a history and narration of who we're as a people. It's told through history with various abstracts of society which include beliefs, clothing, practices and food. What better time for these traditions to be passed down from generation to generation, share rich family recipes, customs, and stories.

Ensuring that the rich tapestry of family heritage is cherished and celebrated. These rituals create a sense of identity and belonging, grounding family members in their roots and strengthening their connection to their cultural heritage.

In addition, family meal time provide an opportunity to teach children social skills and table manners. From learning how to engage in polite conversation to practicing good table etiquette, children acquire essential life skills that extend beyond the dining table. These skills will serve them well in social settings, as they learn to respect others, take turns, and practice good table manners.

A lot of parents struggle to correct their kids today on the littlest of things. With an increasing population of kids by default configuration, wrong mindset and manners to lots of day to day activities. It's now a question of not how but when will we realize to implement the 'catch them while their young' protocol. Being able to have mature healthy conversation with your kids while they're still young and influence them positively as you want to is not only an underrated gift. Its blessings. And the chunk and much of it lays in Family meal time, utilities it.

The benefits of family meal time further extend beyond the physical and social realms. It also has a positive impact on mental health and overall well-being. The nurturing environment created during these meals allows family members to seek and provide emotional support, express gratitude, and celebrate achievements. It becomes a sanctuary where stress is relieved, and a sense of belonging and love is reinforced.

The period creates an avenue for understanding, negotiation you may say. It creates stress release on the parents who are able to communicate to their kids and to an extent even make them understand their ordeal. You can use the little moment to craftily negotiate time from your demanding kids. Growing up, I can still remember negotiating two to three undisturbed hours with mum in exchange for our favorite meal.

Having the right family meal plan system can allow you interact with your kids on a more mature level, getting them to agree to some bidding and on their own part being able to spend time with their parents which goes a long way in helping their self esteem and mental health.

It's also a sure way to monitor your kids' progress. A meal plan that allows the family settle to eat together, helps you monitor and notice growth and development in your kids, also pick up possible wrongs and worries earlier on. In adolescents, I'd be easier for you to pick up the withdrawal instincts in your young adolescents during meal time.

The best definition of adolescence to me is the time your kids no longer come to you to ask for things they normally used. The parent is the first friend of any child, the child's support, confidante and mirror. They look up to them and ask everything. From the rash growing somewhere odd, or the funny surges in the leg or pain in the stomach, a child would normally run to the parent to ask. By the time, a child no longer feels comfortable to come over to discuss everything with the parent, it should be clear to you, you're no longer parenting a child but an adolescent and hence new parenting measures will need to be put in place.

A right family plan can employ meal times in not only noticing the distressing thoughts and withdrawals in adolescents' minds. It can also serve as a way of getting them to feel better and making yourself approachable to discuss relevant issues like sex and hygiene. Say, for example, a daughter who normally used to be active and loud at meal times you noticed to be quiet, flaky and clutching on to her stomach. It makes it clear to you such a child has probably hit menses and needs someone to talk to. You can also use meal times as an effective way to explain the changes adolescence comes with young kids.

"You should reduce your sugar intake now baby, now that you've hit menses!" Saying this to a daughter for example, helps create a moment where you get to educate your child about menses and puberty. You also find it easy to create a path of confidence and trust in the child so they'll come to you for advices and sex talks rather than the wrong channel (peer group and pornography).

Finally, family meal time emphasizes the importance of time management and prioritization. In our ever growing time demanding world, being able to carve out dedicated time for family can be challenging. To establish regular routines and commitments around family meals, families learn to prioritize their relationships and create space for meaningful connections amidst busy schedules is not something easy. Hence, doing with shows high level of discipline and love than cannot be depreciated.

In conclusion, family meal time is not just about the act of eating together; it is a precious opportunity for families to come together, connect, and nurture their relationships. It promotes communication, strengthens bonds, encourages healthy habits, preserves cultural traditions, teaches social skills, enhances mental well-being, and underscores the value of family relationships. So, let us cherish these moments and make family meal time a cherished tradition in our own lives.

# Chapter Three

*Challenges You're Sure to Encounter*

# CHAPTER THREE


As good and important as having a good family meal plan is, it's important to note, it's not without challenges. Some of those challenges include time constraints, busy schedules, work commitments, and extracurricular activities can make it difficult for family members to find a common time to gather for meals. Conflicting schedules and limited time can pose a challenge to consistent family meal times.

Also lack of prioritization, some families may prioritize individual activities or external commitments over shared meal times. The lack of emphasis on the importance of family meals can result in missed opportunities for connection and bonding. There must be commitment to family meal time, there's no two way about it.

Technology distractions. Technology as good as it is has evolved a terrible threat with many adverse consequences. The prevalence of Smartphone, tablets, and other digital devices can distract family members during meal times. Engaging with screens rather than with each other can hinder meaningful conversations and interactions. One would have to strive for face to face interaction over technology.

Meal preparation and planning. The task of planning, shopping for ingredients, and preparing meals can be time-consuming and demanding. The pressure to provide nutritious and appealing meals can be challenging for busy parents or caregivers.

Conflicting dietary preferences of different family members may have varying dietary preferences, restrictions, or allergies. This can make it challenging to plan and prepare meals that cater to everyone's needs and preferences.

**Lack of communication skills.** Lacking effective communication is vital during family meal times. However, family members may struggle with active listening, expressing themselves, or engaging in meaningful conversations. Communication barriers can hinder the quality of interactions during meals.

External influencing factors such as peer pressure, social commitments, or cultural norms may affect family meal times. External influences can make it challenging to maintain consistent family meal traditions or prioritize shared meals.

Existing family dynamics and conflicts is another factor than can impact and hinder the atmosphere during meal times. Tension, unresolved issues, or strained relationships can create a challenging environment for open and positive interaction

# Chapter Four

*Possible Solutions To the Challenges...*

# CHAPTER FOUR
*Possible Solutions To the Challenges...*

While Family Meal Planning does have challenges, it's not away free of solutions. Some solutions to the problems are as follows

**Establishing a regular schedule and keeping to it.** A good meal plan should be well scheduled and consistent. And though it can be hectic, the act itself is a mental exercise that boosts the ability to use time efficiently. Set aside specific days and times each week for family meals. Consistency in scheduling can help family members plan and prioritize their time accordingly.

**Creating a technology-free zone.** Designate the dining area as a screen-free zone during meal times. Encourage family members to put away their devices and focus on engaging with each other. This should not only focus on kids but on other family members as well. Kids are natural emulators. They copy things around them. So instructing your kids not to use phones while using them yourself is to say prolonging a disaster that's still going to happen. Be the role model and explain to the why it's important to have their phones out of interrupting family times.

Also you can capitalize on technology to create hilarious and encouraging reminders to bring the family closer during meals, rather than more distant.

**Involve everyone in meal planning process.** A good meal plan is not a one man work. It's all family members in meal planning and decision-making. Discuss preferences, dietary needs, and explore new recipes together. This promotes a sense of ownership and increases the likelihood of enjoyable meals for everyone. It also increases the percentage possibility of your meal plan to be a success. You don't have to be so tacky about it. Creativity, jokes and flexibility are needed. Be quick enough in stealing moments the families are most close together to eat rather than making a compulsory time for the family meals.

**Sharing meal preparation responsibilities and tasks among family members to alleviate the burden on a single individual.** You might consider assigning age-appropriate tasks to children to foster their involvement and sense of responsibility. Making it a game or something fun can help. This also helps in packing your kids with cooking and time management skills.

**Encourage open communication.** A supportive and non-judgmental environment where family members can openly express themselves during meal times can be your ticket to making it work. Make meal time places where everyone can express themselves actively listen, respect conversations and opinions. And, the sharing of thoughts, experiences, and emotions. If your kids keep feeling loved and respected at a table. They'll definitely come back to that table.

**Embrace flexibility.** Be flexible enough to recognize that family meal times may not always be perfect or go as planned. Embrace flexibility and adapt to changing schedules or unexpected circumstances while still prioritizing regular shared meals. Understand that it won't go smooth as planned. It won't be easy, and it won't be a quick process. You'll require patience, effort, wisdom, flexibility, creativity (and prayer even).

**Make your meal plan it fun and engaging.** Find creative ways to make family meal times enjoyable and engaging. Incorporate games, storytelling, or themed nights to create a lively and memorable dining experience for all ages, genders and preference.

**Seek support from each other.** There's a popular African

proverb that says 'it's both hands that bathe the body'. A meal plan cannot succeed if one person is upholding it and the other tearing down. Family members can support one another by actively participating in conversations, showing interest in each other's lives, and providing emotional support. Encourage an atmosphere of acceptance, understanding, and empathy.

You might need to speak to your partner or husband if you're lady trying to create an active meal plan for your kids.

**Emphasize the importance of family meals to the family members.** Communicate the value and benefits of family meal times to all family members. Don't suffocate them with it. Avoid making them stressed or bugged by your regard for it. Help them understand how shared meals contribute to their overall well-being, relationships, and family unity.

# CONCLUSION

In conclusion, the effective family meal plan is not merely about the act of eating together but encompasses the intentional gathering of family members to share a meal and meaningful conversation. It is a time to foster communication, connection, and bonding among family members.

Family meal time holds significant importance in promoting various positive aspects for both individuals and the family as a whole. It serves as a platform for open discussions, sharing experiences, and building relationships. Through regular family meals, communication is strengthened, creating a supportive and understanding environment within the family unit.

Moreover, family meal times promote healthier eating habits as families plan and prepare nutritious meals together. They provide an opportunity to pass on cultural traditions, family values, and teach children social skills and table manners. The emotional well-being of family members is nurtured as they seek and provide support, express gratitude, and celebrate achievements during meal times.

The effective family meal plan also emphasizes the importance of time management and prioritizing family relationships. By establishing regular routines and appointments, families learn to make time for each other despite busy schedules, thereby strengthening their bonds.

In a world where time and distractions can often pull families apart, the family meal plan becomes a powerful tool to bring them together. It is a chance to create lasting memories, build strong connections, and lay the foundation for a harmonious and loving family environment.

By understanding the significance of family meal time and implementing strategies to overcome challenges, families can reap the numerous benefits it offers. The effective family meal plan is not just about nourishing the body with good food but nourishing the soul with love, togetherness, and shared experiences that will resonate for a lifetime.